IF

THERE

ARE

ANY

HEAVENS

Also by Nicholas Montemarano

The Senator's Children
The Book of Why
If the Sky Falls
A Fine Place

IF

THERE

ARE

ANY

HEAVENS

A Memoir

Nicholas Montemarano

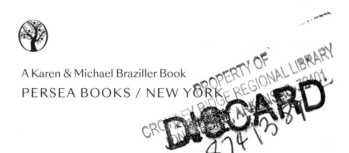

A Karen & Michael Braziller Book
PERSEA BOOKS / NEW YORK

Acknowledgments

(Page numbers refer to the position of the quotations in *If There Are any Heavens*.)

"Listen / with the night falling we are saying thank you" (p. 37) is quoted from "Thanks," from *Migration: New and Selected Poems* by W. S. Merwin (Copper Canyon Press, 2005).

"Naomi underneath this grass" (p.150) and "Lord Lord Lord caw caw caw Lord" (p. 151) are quoted from "Kaddish," from *The Essential Ginsberg* by Allen Ginsberg (HarperCollins 2015).

"If there are any heavens, my mother will(all by herself)have/one" (pp. v and 37), "suddenly in sunlight" (p. 148), and "the whole garden will bow" (p. 148) are quoted from "If there are any heavens, my mother will(all be herself)have" from *Complete Poems 1904–1962* by E. E. Cummings (Liveright, 2016).

Requests for permission to reprint or to make copies and for any other information, should be addressed to the publisher:

Permissions Department
Persea Books
90 Broad Street
New York, NY 10004
Email: permissions@perseabooks.com

Library of Congress Cataloging-in-Publication Data is available upon request.

Hardcover ISBN: 978-0-89255-557-4
E-book ISBN: 978-0-89255-561-1

Design and composition by Rita Lascaro
Typeset in Adobe Jenson Pro
Printed in the United States of America on acid-free paper.

First Edition

if there are any heavens my mother will(all by herself)have one.

—E. E. CUMMINGS

Be not afraid

this is not a poem
though why should a poem
frighten you
words can be oxygen
if that weren't a metaphor
I would inject this not-poem
into my mother
I tell you be not afraid
now will you tell me the same.
/

For most of the worst year

I told my parents how many times

be careful

be safe

keep being safe

wear a mask

wash your hands

please be safe

I know the kids in the neighborhood love

to hug you

but a hug could kill

save the hugs for next year

and they stayed home

didn't attend Mass for a year

rare trip to CVS

grocery store

my mother to get her hair done

post office to mail Christmas gifts

and they washed their hands

and wore masks

but—

/

It began with a cough

that traveled over the phone
from Indiana to Pennsylvania
on Christmas Eve Eve
near the end of the year
people called the worst
just one cough
about which I asked
what was that
because I didn't like its rattle
to which my mother replied
just a cold
even though in the worst year
there was no such thing
as just a cold.
/

People want to know

how

where

who

my sister and I wracked our brains

trying to figure out *how*

maybe a hug from one of the kids

maybe my mother's mask was too loose

but the truth is

we'll never know

we'll never know

we'll never know

and though we wanted desperately

to know

wanted to point to this or that moment

and say there

right *there* and *then*

that's *when* and *how*

we found no answers

that made sense

no *who* or *when* or *where* or *how*

and we will never know

and at a certain point

it no longer mattered.

/

I tried to believe

just a cold
even with more coughing and wheezing
we spoke on Christmas
and she sounded fine
maybe not fine but okay
but later that day a fever
my sister said *shit*
a word she rarely says
shit
and the panic in that word
came through the phone
from her to me
and now we knew what it was
what it had to be
in the year everyone knew was the worst
what we had feared
would find us
had found us
rather had found our mother
and so a rapid test

(positive)
and chest X-ray
(pneumonia)
and our mother was sent home
with steroids and Z-Pak
the way the very sick but not yet critical
are sent home to get better
on their own
or not
and what about our father
(heart disease / diabetes / obesity)
should he move in with my sister
(surely he already had it)
but we couldn't leave our mother alone
so maybe one could live
on one side of the house
the other on the other side
though they used the same bathroom
the same kitchen
breathed the same air
and sure enough the next day
our father felt gunky and exhausted

no interest in food

congested and coughing

had a fever (*shit*)

his muscles so weak

he had trouble standing from a chair

and my sister (a nurse) bought them a pulse oximeter

and said anything below 90

call me immediately

I don't care if it's the middle of the night

I'll sleep with my phone by my ear

and that night

or maybe it was the next

I remember those first days as one long day

our father couldn't get up from the couch

and called to our mother for help

and she pushed and pulled

but he kept falling back

and she said hold on hold on

and hurried to the bathroom to vomit

then back to our father

to push and pull some more

until finally he was up on his feet

hurrying to the bathroom himself
and these were the final days
of the year people called the worst.
/

Breathe: a chorus

If I get corona
I get corona
at the end of the day
I'm not gonna let it stop me
from partying.
/
It's really messing up with my spring break
what is there to do here
other than go to the bars or the beach
and they're closing all of it
I think they're blowing it way out of proportion.
/
We need a refund
this virus ain't that serious
there's more serious things out there.
/
Whatever happens
happens.
/
I just turned 21 this year

so I'm here to party
I mean it sucks
but we're going to make the best of it
I'm from New Orleans
so this really sucks
we're just trying to roll with it
we're just living for the moment
we're just going to let what happens happen.
/
You literally cannot mandate somebody
to wear a mask
knowing that mask
is literally killing people
we the people
are waking up
and every single one of you
that are obeying the devil's laws
is going to be arrested
for crimes against humanity.
/
Are you gonna be a Chinese slave
for the rest of your life

when are you gonna take the mask off
you look like a Chinese slave
when are you gonna take the mask off.
/
It's against the law
to make you wear a mask
it's against the law
you cannot make people wear a mask
this is just made up by Bill Gates
and them
and by you wearing that
seriously think about it
you breathe out your toxic air
then breathe it back in
and you kill your antibodies
you make yourself sick
breathe
no baby
go look on the package
and it will tell you
it will not protect you
from Covid-19

you are hurting yourself
I believe there's a virus
but it's not what they say
we all have viruses
we all get colds
you're being lied to.
/
I'm perfectly healthy
and I don't want to wear a mask
I'm 100% healthy
you just wanna wear a mask
for the rest of your fucking life.
/
People won't learn
these people won't learn
you're a bunch of idiots wearing masks
you know it's not real
look at you fools
you got a fucking doily on your face
you retard
you look like you fucking got it
off your mom's countertop

you look like an idiot
look at you
what are you gonna do
come outside
come outside and show me
how tough you are
I'll beat that fucking mask
off your face
fucking pussy
you're all a bunch of pussies
with your masks.
/
Don't tell me what the fuck to do
how's that pal
use your fucking head
if you know how
you little pimply little shit
you little pimp
I'll leave the store ok.
/
Fuck you where you breathe.
/

This was going to end

one of four ways

    1 my mother and father alive

    2 my mother alive

       but my father dead

    3 my father alive

       but my mother dead

    4 both my mother and father—

but I focused on

hoped for

prayed for

outcome one

both alive

feeling awful for a few weeks

then recovering

just as my sister and her family

had felt awful

but recovered

first my younger niece

who caught Covid

we assume

at her high school
then my sister
fever and vomiting
aches and chills
headaches and dizziness
chest tightness
then her husband
coughing fatigue chills
lightheadedness
shortness of breath
then my older niece
just home from college
for winter break
fever congestion dizziness
days and nights
sleeping the virus away
that was November
that was Thanksgiving
now it was December
Christmas
then the week after
my parents sick

then sicker
one of four outcomes
as the world counted down
the final days of the year.
/

The last email I sent my mother

at the end of that year
included links to movies
I knew she loved
The Best Years of Our Lives
The Bishop's Wife
Duel in the Sun with Jennifer Jones
(after whom my twin sister was named)
A Tree Grows in Brooklyn
which is also my mother's favorite book
she gave me a used first-edition hardback
cracked spine / no dust jacket
what booksellers might call fair
but I would call perfect
a note in the same elegant cursive
she'd used to sign my homework
when I was a boy
Dear Nick
Happy 26th!
This is your first vintage—hope I can find more.
Like this "tree" you're struggling now,

but it will only make you stronger.
Love,
Mom

(I can't recall why I had been struggling
only that I was in grad school and anxious)
my mother responded to my email
thanks a lot love all those movies
will pick a movie and sit in the recliner and watch it
I should make clear: my mother slept in a recliner
by a window in the computer room
and my father slept sometimes on the couch
sometimes in a chair in another room
which they called the Glendale Room
because when they retired and moved
from Glendale Queens to Nappanee Indiana
they wanted one room in Indiana
to remind them of Glendale
same couch / chair / TV / lamps / knick-knacks
even my sister's stuffed koala
whose name was Koala
and who for years we all treated
as if it were alive

this room an attempt at time travel
it could be twenty thirty forty years ago
my mother hadn't wanted to leave New York
her mother was buried there
so was her aunt (her second mother)
there would be no one to visit
their graves
how could she move so far away
from all she had ever known
but my father was tired of New York
tired in general
only a year removed from bypass
and my sister lived in Indiana
where her husband was from
and my parents could be near their grandchildren
so my mother went
reluctantly at first
but grew into their new home
and new routines
and became happy there
doing grandmotherly things
and rescuing stray cats

and praying an hour every morning
starting at 4:30am
a typed four-page list
of people she knew
or had met once
or had never met
but had heard about their troubles
the Glendale Room helped my mother
feel a sense of home
even though she was very far
from the only homes she had known
but whenever I visited
I rarely went in that room
it was too clearly a reproduction
and couldn't convince me
that I was anywhere but Indiana
point is: my father sometimes slept there
in a chair
more often on the couch
my mother on a recliner
on the other side of the house
their bodies uncomfortable in their bed

and now at the end of the worst year

as I tried to sleep

in Pennsylvania

I imagined them sleeping

or not

in Indiana

my mother wheezing in a chair

my father coughing on the couch

getting up three four five times in the night

to pee

his walker (hip surgery) tapping against the floor

so I sent my mother links to movies

she could play on the computer

within view of the chair

where she spent her days and nights

in and out of fever-aches

and fever-chills

with her lungs trying to do their work

and the virus doing its work

and silly me I thought old movies

would help.

/

Never got to watch those movies

because the next day
the last day of the year people called the worst
my sister took our parents together
for monoclonal antibody infusions
lab-made proteins dripped into their bodies
to do battle with the virus
I would like to think it was romantic
this infusion date
but my father could hardly walk
even with his walker
and during the ride home
my mother was trembling with chills
so my sister dropped off my father
and took my mother home with her
where her fever spiked to 103
and her hands shook so much
she couldn't bring a pill or cup of water to her mouth
and my sister texted me: *shit call me now!*
and when I did: *this is bad / this is really bad*
her voice shaking

she took our mother to an urgent care center
where they took a chest X-ray
(double-pneumonia)
and checked her oxygen
(84)
and said *you need to go to the nearest ER*
immediately
before this my mother had said
no hospitals / I'm not going
no one likes hospitals
but my mother especially not
she was extremely claustrophobic
and knew she'd have to get on an elevator
(she hadn't stepped on one in fifty years
walked up fourteen flights in the hospital
to see my father after his bypass:
don't worry I'll take the stairs slow
I'll stop to rest every few floors)
plus there was the Covid narrative:
if you go to a hospital
you never go home
my sister wanted our mother at the best hospital

which happened not to be the closest
so she signed a release
in case our mother didn't survive
that she had been advised to go to the closest ER
but went against that advice
and drove our mother to a hospital farther away
my mother didn't understand
why they weren't stopping home
to pick up clothes and a few other things
and my sister explained
that there was no time for that
and during the ride to the ER our mother shook
and upon arrival they took her oxygen
(still 84)
and brought her a wheelchair
and just like that wheeled her away
from my sister
who sat in the parking lot
for the next six hours
texting back and forth with our mother
already knowing that she would be admitted
but not leaving until she was in a room

meanwhile here in Pennsylvania
I received a frantic call from my father
he was stuck in a chair at home
had been stuck hours and hours
couldn't get up
was soaked with sweat
where did everyone go
where's your sister and your mother
I keep calling but no one answers
I tried to explain what was happening
but my father dropped his phone
then his voice as if from a great distance
fucking chair for fucking six hours
he didn't sound like him
not things he would say
or how he would say them
and I worried that his own fever had spiked
and he was confused
and I kept saying
Dad! Dad! Dad!
can you hear me Dad
but his voice receded

I can't get up / what am I supposed to do
I hung up and called my sister
who called her husband
to get our father out of the chair
and this is how the final hours
of the final day
of the year people called the worst
ended.
/

Everything became about oxygen

how much extra my mother needed
to keep her oxygen saturation stable (95+)
and when her O2 sat became unstable
how much more my mother needed
three liters per minute from a nasal cannula
became six liters per minute
became a high-flow nasal cannula
at 45%
at 55%
at 85%
she was as her doctor said
not moving in the right direction
sometimes when we spoke on the phone
she sounded weak and short of breath
but other times better
just tired
my wife texted her photos of our son
and during our calls I kept saying
you're doing great
just keep resting

do your breathing exercises
do you think you can get on your stomach
that's supposed to be good
we can ask the nurses to turn you over
(she said it hurt her back too much)
well if you can't prone
then maybe spend some time on your side
can you turn onto your side
we'll have the nurses get you on your side
she said that her room's door was closed
(every door on the Covid unit had to be closed)
and the nurses were so nice
and she wasn't interested in TV
she was fine with peace and quiet
no appetite
just very thirsty
once she said
if it's my time it's my time
and I know she meant this
though she kept breathing
into her incentive spirometer
and was proud when she coughed up mucus

the doctors said she wasn't getting worse

but wasn't getting better

and was needing a lot of oxygen

and listen we've seen patients in your mom's condition

recover and go home

but not very often

let's just wait and see.

/

Just stay calm

this is a flu
this is like a flu
it's a little like a regular flu
we lose thousands and thousands of people a year
to the flu
life and the economy go on
we don't turn the country off
you know a lot of people think
this goes away with the heat
we've done a pretty good job
it's going to disappear
one day like a miracle
you know it could get worse
before it gets better
it could maybe go away
we'll see what happens
nobody really knows
you have to be calm
we're prepared
and we're doing a great job with it

and it will go away

and we're going to have a great victory

it's going to go away

hopefully at the end of the month

and if not

hopefully soon after that

it's going to go

it's going to leave

it's going to be gone

it's going to be eradicated

it's going to pass

this virus is going to disappear

it's a question of when

you know nobody knew anything

now we know

we can put out fires

we're not going to see it again

hopefully

after a period of time

eventually it's going to be gone

it may flare up

and it may not flare up

we'll have to see what happens
at some point this stuff goes away
it's going to work out fine
people are getting better
they're all getting better
it's dying out
we're very close to therapeutics
but I don't even like to talk about that
because it's fading away
it's dying out
the numbers are starting to get very good
and I think we are going to be very good
I'll be right eventually
I'll say it again
it's going to disappear and I'll be right
we're going to beat it
I say it's going to disappear
and they say oh that's terrible
well it's true
I mean it's going to disappear
I think we can knock it out
it will go away like things go away

absolutely no question in my mind
hopefully sooner rather than later
and frankly you know
we've had a tremendous market
and you and I have talked about that
the stock market
think of it
we're almost back to where we were
and they scream how can you say that
we have vaccines coming
we have therapeutics coming
and you'll see
the pandemic goes away
once you get to a certain number
you know we use the word herd right
once you get to a certain number
it's going to go away
the vaccine will end the pandemic
but it's ending anyway
I mean they go crazy when I say it
it's going to peter out
and it's going to end

but we're going to help the end
it's gonna run its course
it's gonna end
they'll go crazy
watch it'll be a headline tomorrow
these people are crazy
no it's running its course
it happens
people have it and it goes
what happens is you get better
that's what happens
you get better
and then you're immune
we are rounding the final turn
there has to be a calmness
you don't want me jumping up and down
screaming
there's going to be great death
nobody would have ever thought
a thing like this
could have happened.
/

January 6, 2021

will be remembered
by most people
as the day Trump terrorists
stormed and penetrated the U.S. Capitol
but for me
it's the day my sister called:
You need to come now
the doctor said we need to come
I wandered around the house
confused and afraid and almost useless
while my wife and son
made me sandwiches for the ride
and packed food for the hotel
hard-boiled eggs and yogurt and granola
and cold-brew coffee
and packed my clothes and snow boots
and of course many masks
I showered and got dressed
and packed my computer and chargers
then the usually hard decision

which books to bring
I had no interest in anything
except getting out the door and on the road
but always bring books wherever I go
I was about to reread *Death of a Salesman*
(not that)
I was reading Beckett's short fiction
(absolutely not)
I stared at the spines of my favorites
but my reading taste buds were dead
then I remembered that Cummings poem
if there are any heavens my mother will(all by herself)have
one
and put his *100 Selected Poems* in my bag
and then remembered my favorite Merwin
Listen / with the night falling we are saying thank you
and put one of his books in my bag
and finally my Bible
O Lord heal me for my bones are troubled
I am weary with my moaning
by the car I hugged my wife and son
knowing that no matter what happened

I wouldn't return the same person
and then I drove
through a long cold dreary day and night
early in the new year
that was supposed to be better
than the previous one
I turned on the radio now and then
to feel less alone
only to feel more alone
everything was news about the Capitol
but (forgive me) I didn't care
if democracy lived or died
not then
I couldn't think much except
my mother is dying
I'm driving ten hours to see my mother
who is dying
then: maybe not
maybe she'll get better
right now she's still alive
I drove through Pennsylvania
then endless empty Ohio

stopping at rest stops to pee
steering clear of unmasked people
or those whose noses were exposed
washing and washing my hands
pumping gas
disinfecting my hands
eating a hard-boiled egg
I stopped sometimes to take a call
from my sister with updates
oxygen levels
blood work
inflammation markers
what the nurse said
what the doctor said
and to call my wife
tell her where I was
how I was
though I had words only for where
not how
and I stopped once in the dark
to call my mother
to say I was on my way

to ask how she was

was she eating

was she resting

was she in the bed or the chair

was she doing her breathing exercises

be there soon

see you soon

I love you

then a few more hours

until Ohio became Indiana.

/

How strange

to be in a room
in a mostly empty hotel
ten minutes from my mother
maybe dying
how strange to be in a hotel at all
for the first time in a year
I wiped down every surface
that could be wiped
toilet / room phone / remote control / light switches
I stared at the bed for a long time
before sitting on it
it was 11pm and I was exhausted from driving
but afraid to turn out the lights
and close my eyes
I lay in bed and prayed
by which I mean talked to God
asking for strength
but not for God to save my mother
I believe in the power of prayer
and in miracles

(*let this cup pass from me*)
but know from life experience
what one asks for
one doesn't always get
(*yet not as I will but as you will*)
so it didn't feel right to ask God
to spare my mother
when my mother's life
was and had always been in God's hands
better I thought to ask for strength
whatever may come
especially in the morning
when I would see my mother.
/

End of life

my sister told me I had to say
those three words
I'm here for an end-of-life visit with my mother
I said to the woman who greeted me
inside the hospital
I had sat in the parking garage
for ten minutes
taking deep breaths
and crying
and trying not to cry
before putting on my mask
and walking to the entrance
knowing I had to say
end of life
a few days earlier my mother had texted me
went downstairs to main lobby for chest X-ray
took two elevators would you believe
down and up
now I'm having apple juice and a nap
talk to you later

to which I replied

wow two elevators you're becoming a pro

have a nice nap

please rest

we're going to see if there's a way

to get you on your stomach

for a little bit

without pain in your back

hang in there

rest easy

take deep breaths

and know that Jen and I are on the case

my mother:

hi my phone was charging

got your voicemail

have been resting off and on

in the recliner

I texted her photos of my son

and pep-talked her

one day at a time

one breath at a time

keep doing what you're doing

my mother:
thank you
love you
when I talked with her during the drive
she had sounded tired
but not *end of life*
whatever that sounds like
I'm no doctor
and my mother's numbers
were her numbers
and now after ten hours of driving
and a night of little sleep
and a cup of hotel room coffee
and a short drive through a cold gray Indiana morning
and ten minutes in the parking garage
praying for strength
I was saying the words
end of life
to a woman who seemed to be expecting me
she had my name on a piece of paper
took my temperature
asked me the usual Covid screening questions

asked me to take off my mask

and put it into my pocket

gave me a new mask to wear

asked me to sit in the waiting area

for a chaplain to escort me up

to see my mother.

/

At the nurses' station

right outside my mother's room (6107)

its door closed

all the doors closed

a nurse helped with my gown

tied the straps around the back

gave me another new mask

told me to put the old new mask

they'd given me in the lobby

in my pocket

gave me rubber gloves

told me to tuck the sleeves of my gown

into the gloves

gave me goggles that covered my glasses

said I'd have an hour

take a little longer if you need
no rush
the nurse told me exactly what to do
when it was time to leave
first tear off the gown inside the room
tear it just like the Hulk
then remove the gloves
toss all that into the trash
disinfect your hands at the door
leave the goggles on until you're out
but if you forget any of that
the nurse said
just press the call button
and we'll come in to help
I had only half-listened
and already knew I'd need to call the nurse
when it was time to go
I stood outside the room
unsure what to do
the nurse said I could go in
there would be a chair beside my mother's
she was excited to see me.

/

Breathing oxygen through a nasal cannula
my mother sat in a recliner
the last time I saw her
she was 79 years old
but now looked closer to 85
her breathing slightly labored
but she was awake and alert and happy
to see me
I leaned over her
and reached my arms around her
and through my mask
kissed her head.
/
Because it wasn't easy for her to speak
I spoke
how happy I was to see her
how proud of her I was
two elevator rides
after so many years of none
I tried to get her on an elevator once
it will be over in seconds Mom
trust me you'll be fine

but she rather would have died
than step foot on it
(childhood trauma from being locked in a cellar
by mean girls in her neighborhood)
here at the hospital they'd drugged her
before wheeling her onto the elevator
she hardly remembered it
but I was proud anyway
strange that I don't remember much else
we talked about that hour
I just remember being positive
reassuring her that Jen and I were *on the case*
sleuths trying to solve the mystery
of how to save her
I remember telling her that if I had my way
I'd carry her out of the hospital
that was the fantasy that had popped
into my head
over and over
lifting my mother into my arms
and carrying her home
the room was dark and small

the virus sealed away from anyone not in the room
on a small table beside the recliner was my mother's phone
and a chocolate chip cookie wrapped in plastic
and a white plastic cup filled with orange juice
which my mother sipped through a straw
because her mouth was so dry
I kept telling her rest
just take care of you
Jen and I are on this
we're talking to the nurses and doctors every day
we'll handle everything
don't worry about a thing
just keep doing your breathing exercises
and coughing up what you can
(while I was there she coughed up mucus
and I said good that's good
and remembered how hard it was for me and my sister
to cough up mucus when we were kids
our mother slapping our backs
even sticking her finger down our throats
saying there you go good get it up
and once the two of us shivering naked in a tub

with high fevers while our mother washed our bodies
with rubbing alcohol)
two of her lower teeth were hers
the bridge between them probably in a case in her bag
and this made her seem older
but the way she breathed with two quick inhales
it was impossible to look at her
without thinking: my mother is very sick
I could see that she was getting tired
and said that I would let her rest
and kissed her again through my mask
and rubbed her back and shoulders
and she said oh that feels nice
and I told her that I loved her
and would call her later
that I'd be there every day if I could
I pressed my mother's call button
and the nurse came in and told me to tear off my gown
and pull off my gloves
and throw those away inside the room
but leave on my goggles and mask
I did exactly what he said

then said see you Mom

I love you

see you soon

not knowing if I would ever

see her again

and disinfected my hands on the way out

and once in the hallway removed my goggles

and replaced the mask I'd been wearing

with one from my pocket

and took the elevator to the ground floor

and walked out of the hospital

and into the parking garage

and sat in my car

and wept

before driving to see my father.

/

My father sat in an armchair

that had been moved from the living room
into the kitchen
so that he could brace himself
on the kitchen table
and use his arm strength
to push himself up out of the chair
his legs were too weak
to get him up from the couch
so he spent all day and night
in this chair
except when using his walker
to walk to the bathroom
on the table was a thermometer
a blood pressure cuff
the same pulse oximeter my mother had used
before she was hospitalized
my father had lost weight
when I arrived he put on a mask
because I was the only one in our family
not to have had Covid

I wore a mask of course
and sat on the sofa in the living room
about twenty feet from him
I had to ask him to turn down the TV
so I could hear him
and he could hear me
then it seemed ridiculous
sadly so
that a son should need to sit so far away
from his father
whose wife might be dying
so I carried a chair from the dining room
closer to my father
but still ten feet away
he told me he was tired
very tired
and had no interest in food
was listless
I told him about my time with my mother
and that she was needing more and more oxygen
the worry was what would happen
when there was no more oxygen to give

my mother had said no ventilator
had been clear about that
we talked about people we knew
or people we knew who knew people
who had been on a ventilator for weeks
and were still alive
or had made it home
but she doesn't want that
I told my father
and he shook his head
as if to say: what are we supposed to do
or: how did this happen / how did we get to this place
I fed their cat and gave it water
then fed the stray cats outside
that my mother had been feeding
for years
dozens of cats
some named some not
only weeks ago my mother had told me
that she had found a sick kitten beside the house
so sick she knew it was dying
and she carried it into her garage

where it was warmer
and wrapped the kitten in a towel
and sat in a chair and held the kitten
until it passed
I helped my father make a grocery list
offered to get him anything he needed
drove recycling to the recycling center
then with my brother-in-law took down
the Christmas decorations on the lawn
trees and snowmen and yards and yards of lights
we wound around our arms
and carried down to the basement
I stayed with my father until almost dark
sports and movies muted on TV
and texted with my sister
what the nurse said
why hadn't the doctor called back
what my doctor friend in PA had said
what her respiratory therapist friend had said
what we had looked up online
how could we get our mother to prone
what were her latest numbers

how much oxygen was she on at night
how much during the day
and what did that mean
then I drove back to the hotel
ten minutes from my mother
who I couldn't see
I stopped at a nearby supermarket
to buy yogurt and rolls and cheese and turkey
even though I've been vegetarian for twenty-five years
because I don't know why
maybe because my body wanted protein
and was too tired to resent the man at checkout
not wearing a mask
and back in the hotel lobby bar
I ordered a drink
I wanted something with bourbon
which I would normally sip straight
but for some reason asked for an old fashioned
and the bartender
a young woman who bless her wore her mask correctly
had to look up how to make one
it's been a minute since I made one of those

she said

which meant she had never made one

and I regretted my decision

should have asked for a beer

and she messed up the first try

and said sorry let me give that another go

and now I had been standing in the lobby longer

than I had wanted to

and eventually I took the drink and my groceries

up to my room

and wiped the outside of the glass

and even the rim

with a Clorox wipe

and felt paranoid that the virus was on the glass

was everywhere

and threw away the orange wedge

which the bartender had touched with her hands

and drank the drink quickly

(it wasn't good but what did I care)

and then lay in bed

and read Psalms

about suffering and healing

and called my mother to say goodnight
we spoke only briefly because she was tired
and they were getting her ready for bed
I told her that it was important for her
to keep the CPAP on during the night
to try not to take it off
they would give her something for anxiety
but it was important to get that oxygen
through the night
I told her
and she said I love you
and I said I love you
and then I was alone in a hotel room
in Elkhart Indiana
with no interest in TV or reading or sleep
and I thought of my father
sleeping in the chair in the kitchen
or not sleeping
and what else was I to do now
but turn out the lights
get into bed
pray some more

sleep an hour here

an hour there

and wait for whatever the next day would bring.

/

Wait and see: a chorus

DOCTOR
Here's what I see:
she's gotten all the care we can offer
antibody preparation
outpatient Z-Pak
steroids and remdesivir
she's currently semi-stable
i.e. >24 hours at the edge
of respiratory failure
despite all appropriate treatments
some things got worse on the 5th
her inflammation and oxygen demands went up that day
she's clearly said to the doctors
not to intubate her
I think this is appropriate
as ventilation hasn't improved people's chances
of walking out of the hospital
she should have been told a million times now
to prone as much as possible
get a bean bag / get the right face sponge / get her
    comfy face down

if she worsens from here
meaning she can't keep her oxygen up
despite current support
and if your family can find the will and the way
you can consider having her at home
as she passes with hospice care
I have seen people return from this edge
just not many
and not over 55
if she has to be on CPAP continuously
it's time to consider home or hospice
where you and your brother can be with her
I'm sorry your family is going through this
let me know what questions you might have.

JEN
So you think her numbers
most likely will not improve
are you saying timewise
she may have
only 24 hours
should we make a full-court press

have her wear the CPAP
as much as possible
prone for the next 24 hours
then get her hospice home care
are her lungs just shot.

DOCTOR
Covid has obliterated her ability to oxygenate
her blood effectively
through lung tissue inflammation
and infection damage
unsure of the permanence of this
she will get through this or not
depending on the strength of her heart
and prior health of her lungs
we are in a precarious time.

JEN
Maybe if she can make it to tomorrow. . .
no prior heart or lung problems
I think we had false hope last night
when the nurse told me her blood oxygen went up

do we give it another day
see if her numbers trend up.

DOCTOR
I think we wait
until she can't tolerate
any more high-flow nasal cannula
i.e. is only on CPAP
until then she prones as much as possible
takes some deep breaths
and coughs that crap up
and we hope.

ME
Just spoke with Mom
she sounded very good
was still doing breathing exercises
pep-talked her big time about what a great day she had
best I've heard her sound
like before she was sick
she definitely wants to come home
I don't mean tomorrow

but eventually
also told her I hope she has more good days
but that if for some reason she doesn't
not to get down
that it's normal maybe even expected
to have some good days and some not as good
and she said believe me I know
she seems ready for whatever it takes
I said to her
I want nothing more
than for you to walk through the door
of your home
we're doing everything
to make that happen
she said God that would be great
I wouldn't care at all if I needed oxygen
I can't wait to get home.

DOCTOR
I know it's late
I can see where your distress comes from
your mom looks fabulous

is speaking coherently
and yet persists in this critical state
I don't know if she will recover or not
truthfully
but she's trying hard
she's being well-loved
and is in no pain
we talked intubation and hospice
she isn't ready for either
so we wait
these must be long days.

JEN

Not too late
I don't sleep much
I know that despite some things getting a little better
for my mom
her requirements are still awful
she's really fighting
I made inquiries about hospice
because I realize the bottom can drop out
at any time

all so confusing.

DOCTOR

She's not ready for hospice

she's too strong right now

she's showing us strength with her improving labs

her repositioning efforts

her breathing exercises

she'll tell you if she can't fight any longer

long-term prognosis is unclear to me

for lungs that have Covid to this degree

I can imagine her like a patient

with pulmonary fibrosis

on portable oxygen

winded with too long a walk

dodging respiratory viruses as they come

it could be a good life yet

let's wait together and see.

JEN

I just FaceTimed Mom

had a long conversation

she was just kind of talking about everything
so that was nice
I'm a little upset she was in bed all day
never got to the chair
this is a critical time
a body can take only so much
they opened her window today
because it was beautiful and sunny.
/

The only time I ever cried

in front of students
was about my mother
the class was contemporary autobiography
and the prompt was to write about a life
other than your own
from that person's perspective
using that person's words
recording / transcribing / editing them
to make art
an oral history project
think Studs Terkel or Svetlana Alexievich
except this would be one person's story
for example I said
if I ever pursued such a project
it would be about my mother
her story in her words
specifically about her childhood
in Bushwick Brooklyn
how she grew up poor
never knew her father

her mother sick and bedbound
with a heart condition caused by rheumatic fever
both of them supported by my mother's aunt
who worked in an olive cannery
so poor my mother had to beg
the pharmacist for the medication
that kept her mother alive
(sometimes he said no)
she went to school each day afraid
she'd come home to her mother gone
some days the children on her street
would tell her
your mother's dead
we saw them take the body
and my mother would run inside
terrified it was true
no matter how many times
they had tricked her
and as soon as these words left my mouth
my students gasped
one said oh my God
and though I'd heard this story from my mother

I had never told anyone
had never heard the words come out of my mouth
nor heard another's reaction
and only upon hearing my class's response
did I feel the full emotional weight of the story
and my voice stopped
I couldn't go on
I knew that if I tried to say another word
no words would come
I held up my hand as if to say
give me a moment
and then I did say that
or something like it
I'm sorry I need a moment
and waited with the emotions
in my chest and face and eyes
with some students looking at me
but most looking down
bless them
to give me the illusion of privacy
and after a minute
probably not even

I collected myself enough
to give them a writing prompt
but didn't excuse myself to the restroom
stayed where I was
sitting on the desk at the front of the room
eyes closed
listening to them write.
/
Three years after that day
not long before my mother got sick
I felt a strong urge to tell her story
have her tell it in her own words
record / transcribe / shape / midwife it
suddenly it was the most important thing
I could write about
the girl my mother was
in mid-century Brooklyn
born the month before Pearl Harbor
her absent father
the one time she heard him at the door
asking if he could come in to see her
and being told to go away

her father just a name: Matthew

did she ever try to find him

why or why not

what was her mother like

what did she look like

the greatest loss of my mother's life

gone when my mother was only 14

but these questions were too intimate

for the phone

so I decided to wait

until the next time I saw my mother

which would be who knew when

given the virus

maybe not until summer

and now it was the year

that was supposed to be better

than the worst year

and I was living in a hotel

in Elkhart Indiana

my mother in a hospital

ten minutes away

her lungs *obliterated* by a virus

trying hard
sounding better
hoping to return home
but persisting in a critical state.
/

Hallelujah

may seem too strong a word
forgive me
but hallelujah
my mother woke one day
with an appetite
oatmeal with brown sugar
for breakfast
and coffee
just a few sips
but hallelujah coffee
more oatmeal for lunch
and cheesecake
hallelujah a craving for cheesecake
the nurse brought more for dinner
and my mother FaceTimed my father
the first time they saw each other's faces
in this new year
I didn't think my mother or father knew
how to FaceTime
I think my mother hit the button

by accident

but the wrong button turned out to be

the right button

one that cheered my father

who remember was still sick

still not eating much

still exhausted and sleeping in the chair

by the kitchen table

and hallelujah he was so happy

to see her face

his voice changed slightly

I could hear it

not baby talk

but (what to call it) cutesy talk

the voice I remember my father using

with my mother

sometimes

when we were kids

hey Cat he'd say

hey he'd say when he came home from work

hey he'd call out to the house

not how ya doing

in his Brooklynese
but how ya boo-in
hey Cat how ya boo-in
and hallelujah I could hear that voice now
hey look who it is he said
I got Mommy on FaceTime
look at you
you look good
and they talked about oatmeal and cheesecake
and hallelujah coffee
and how he was doing
(still tired / no interest in food)
and they didn't need long
my mother didn't have the energy
maybe ten minutes
but it was nice to hear
from across the room
my father's side
of the conversation
and hallelujah my mother
needed less oxygen
only slightly less

very slightly less
still too much
but less was less
and an appetite was an appetite
praise the Lord coffee
and I watched football with my father
me masked in one room
my father in his chair
and for those three hours we were able
not to forget
which would be impossible
but set aside
that's the best way to put it
set aside our worry about my mother
set it down just for a few hours
in another room
and watch a football game
get lost I guess in the unfolding drama
of a playoff game
and when I got thirsty
I went into the guest bedroom
where I stay with my wife and son

whenever we visit

and where neither my mother nor father

had been in weeks

and which was or felt safe

and where I kept my coat and bag and water bottle

and once in that room I removed my mask

and drank water

and opened a window

to breathe cold fresh air

before rejoining my father

and then my sister came

and her husband

and their oldest daughter

and they all wore masks

even though they'd already had the virus

just in case

and we all watched football

and if this had been some other Sunday

my wife and son would be watching with us

and my mother would be in the kitchen

maybe cleaning (neatest person I've ever known)

or getting a snack for my son

or in the computer room answering emails
or on Facebook liking photos
of the children of children
my sister and I went to grade school with
and photos of the children and grandchildren
of old neighbors from Queens
and the children and grandchildren
of neighbors in Indiana
and praying for anyone
who needed prayers
whether someone she knew or not
and as much as we wanted to believe
this could be any Sunday
in any year
my mother wasn't there
and the same virus
that had been in my sister's body
and her husband's body
and their children's bodies
and was still in my father's body
was in my mother's
but hallelujah oatmeal

it's going to disappear
and hallelujah cheesecake
it's going to go
and hallelujah coffee
it's going to pass
and hallelujah FaceTime
it's going to work out fine
and hallelujah (slightly) less oxygen
the numbers are starting to get very good
and Lord let her need less tomorrow
and I think we are going to be very good
and less the next day
we're going to beat it
and less the day after
we can knock it out
and Lord more oatmeal
it will go away like things go away
and cheesecake
people have it and it goes
and coffee
what happens is you get better
and FaceTime

we are rounding the final turn
and Lord let her one day
however many days from now
walk into this home
and we will sing
we are already singing
hallelujah.
/
That night my son and I watched
the Steelers-Browns playoff game
together: me in a hotel room in Indiana
my son in our home in Pennsylvania
my face on his computer screen
his face on mine
this had been my wife's idea
we had been apart five days
and rarely missed a Steelers game
never a playoff game
even though he was 11
and it was a school night
he was allowed to stay up late
though at first it may seem

beside the point

I should say

that the Steelers started the season 11-0

there was talk of going undefeated

but they lost four of their last five

and limped into the playoffs

a team no good team feared

not even the Browns

though their long-suffering fans

might have felt otherwise

no playoff wins in twenty-six years

and now a Covid outbreak

sidelining four Browns players and their head coach

on the first play from scrimmage

the Steelers center snapped the ball

over the quarterback's head

and it rolled into the end zone

where the Browns recovered

for a touchdown fourteen seconds into the game

four minutes later the Steelers QB

threw an interception

and a minute after that

the Browns scored another touchdown

another interception and two touchdowns later

the Browns were up 28-0

at the end of the first quarter

and by the end of the half

the score was 35-10

a stunning almost certainly unsurmountable lead

it's over

my son and I agreed

we're done

no chance

forget it

can't believe it

no way they come back from this

there are some fans of some teams

who might have given up

and gone to bed

but we're not them

we'll see what happens

nobody really knows

you have to be calm

so we kept watching

kept hoping
despite the odds
and sure enough late in the third quarter
the Steelers started to come back
they scored two touchdowns
and were down only 35-23
the numbers are starting to get very good
with plenty of time left
we're going to have a great victory
and suddenly what had seemed certain
to be one of the worst losses
had a chance to become
one of the greatest comebacks
we're coming back so fast
we'll go crazy
we'll be jumping up and down screaming
it'll be a headline tomorrow
but early in the fourth quarter
the Browns scored again
to go up 42-23
and again it was over
absolutely no chance now

that was the death blow

might as well go to bed

but we didn't

and even as we said done / over / dead

we (secretly) hoped

because you never know

because why not

because stranger things have happened

and sure enough the Steelers scored

to cut the lead to 42-29

not much time left

but maybe

if everything goes exactly right

maybe just enough time

we'll go crazy

we'll be jumping up and down

but then the Browns extended their lead

to 48-29

and now truly absolutely without a doubt

it was over

the game

the season

nobody would have ever thought
a thing like this
could have happened
but we kept watching
and my son said
it doesn't matter that they lost
what matters is that we watched together
and it was so *him* to say this
and I agreed
and the Steelers scored again
to make the score a respectable looking 48-37
but the numbers were deceiving
it had been a rout from the first play
we'd had hope
but in retrospect it had been hopeless
we watched until time expired
and said goodnight
said I love you
and then I was alone in a hotel room
I turned out the lights
and got into bed
and thought of my mother so close

and prayed
Lord let her sleep well
Lord let her breathe better
Lord let her wake craving oatmeal and coffee
Lord let her come home.
/
The next day
my mother did eat
oatmeal and cheesecake
and drank coffee
and when I spoke with her
when I *saw* her
over FaceTime
she didn't seem sick
every conversation we'd had before this
had been five maybe ten minutes
but this one lasted
(I checked the time on my phone)
thirty-three minutes
what happened to your Steelers
she said
and asked how my son was doing in school

and I said are you doing your breathing exercises

keep it up

you're doing great

you look great

we just want to get you home

be patient

recovery can take time

we love you

get some rest

sleep well tonight okay

talk to you tomorrow

love you

bye

love you.

/

I bought my mother an iPad

so that she could watch
Little House on the Prairie
her favorite show
ours too growing up
reruns every day after school
if my mother could watch
her favorite old movies and shows
it would pass the time
would help her feel that much better
my wife said let's buy her an iPad
give her our Amazon Prime password
they have every season of *Little House*
so I ordered one online for pickup at Target
and then sat with my father
while he watched NFL highlights
and I set up the iPad
even started watching the *Little House* pilot
so that when I dropped off the iPad at the hospital
and they bagged it
and brought it up to my mother

she would only need to press play
and could watch all nine seasons
two hundred four episodes
maybe that would help get her through
however many more weeks
she would need to stay
before coming home.
/

But my mother had a rough night

by which the nurse meant
that the CPAP had caused my mother anxiety
despite anti-anxiety meds
and she pulled it off
not sure how many times
and her oxygen dropped
from semi-stable 91 or 92
into the unstable 80s
setting off an alarm
that woke my mother
and the nurse came into the room
not sure how many times
to reaffix the CPAP
and the next day my mother was tired and weak
and sounded sick again
(which of course she still was)
and our conversations were brief
though she did say
it had been a dark and stormy night
and that made us laugh

and maybe convinced us
that a mother who can make a joke
about a bad night
in a hospital
during a pandemic
is a mother strong enough
to keep doing breathing exercises
and cough that crap up
as the doctor had said
and keep trying
to get home
and we kept pep-talking her
that it was *so so so* important
for her to keep the CPAP on
during the night
that the oxygen it pushed into her lungs
was her lifeline
and we asked the nurses what they could do
to make our mother less anxious
more comfortable
maybe change the timing of when she got Xanax
in relation to when they put the CPAP over her face

something / anything
certainly our mother wasn't the first claustrophobe
who needed to wear a CPAP in order to live
certainly they had tricks
things they'd tried with other patients
that had worked
and the nurses explained
that the CPAP had been too tight
so they loosened its straps
but that allowed our mother to pull it off
so they'd give her more Xanax
(though they didn't want to depress
her respiration too much)
and get her as relaxed as possible
before putting on the mask
and maybe they'd put it on a bit later
and my sister said to me
if only they'd let me in the room
I'd make sure she keeps that mask on
and I'd prone her during the day
get her on her stomach and rub her back
they need the help

the next time the doctor called
my sister slipped this into a conversation
I'm a nurse she said
if only I could be in the room
with my mother
but the doctor didn't bite
not even a nibble
so there went that idea
my sister and I were constantly trying
to think of ideas
solutions
things we may not have thought about
were constantly researching
and talking to people
and to each other
about what else we might do
because our mother remained
wait and see
precarious
critical
the hope was for her to come home
I was planning to move in with my parents

for as long as it took

to help care for them

would teach my classes online

from Indiana

but at the same time that I held this hope

in one hand

in the other hand

was hospice

conversations about end of life

how we might bring my mother home

have her spend her final hours

in her own bed

with her family around her

my father

me and Jen

her grandchildren

we knew that was how she'd want

to go

if she had to

but she was already on too much oxygen

to come home

by which the doctors meant

that she wouldn't survive the ambulance ride
with the amount of oxygen an ambulance
is allowed to give
so if
if
we reached a point at which my mother
wouldn't recover
she would have to pass
in the hospital
and after such conversations
and considerations
we were back on the case
me and my sister
twin sleuths looking for a magical
maybe miraculous
something
neither we nor the doctors had tried.
/

The next day

was the first day
we didn't speak with her
none of us
not me or Jen or our father
because she'd had another bad night
and was tired
and wearing the CPAP during the day
to make up for not having worn it
much of the night
but we still looked for hope
of course
and he showed up
in the form of a new doctor
from Johns Hopkins
who might know something
the other doctors didn't
might have some trick up his sleeve
he told us that if our mother had another
bad night
then the next day he would order

a scan that would show

whether or not her lungs

were beyond repair

and though the prospect of knowing

that her lungs would never heal

was frightening

it would be better to know

than not to know

plus (hope) the scan might show

that her lungs could heal

in which case

more breathing exercises

keep the CPAP on at all costs

get her to prone for God's sake

we went to bed that night with a plan

to call the nurse every three hours

my sister at midnight

me at 3am

and so on

shortly after midnight my sister called me

to say that our mother's blood pressure had dropped

and I needed to ask about that at 3:00

and for the next three hours I tried to sleep
but didn't
and when I called the nurse said
that my mother was now on BiPAP
rather than CPAP
because her oxygen had dropped
into the mid-80s
which was not a good sign
and they had given her some morphine
and that word
morphine
I didn't expect that word
didn't know what it meant
not exactly
but as soon as my sister heard that word
from my mouth
she called the nurse
then called me back
and said we need to go now
when can you be at the hospital
so I showered and dressed
and drove through the dark early morning

of Elkhart Indiana

and met my sister in the parking lot

at 4:30am

and together we went inside

and again said those words

we're here for an end-of-life visit

with our mother.

/

Search history

butter sage sauce for ravioli

coronavirus latest map and case count

if you sign up for spotify premium do you lose playlists

barney miller christmas episodes

west wing christmas episodes

cheers christmas episodes

charlie brown christmas

donny marie osmond christmas

insurrection act

wonder woman 1984

how to cook fresh ravioli

radicalism of jesus christ

premier league table

covid mortality rate by age

covid recovery rate in united states by age

covid recovery rate 79 year old

that is solemn we have ended dickinson

coronavirus latest map and case count

pneumonia and coronavirus

disease progression covid pneumonia

mortality covid pneumonia

2020 nfl playoff picture

steelers most likely first-round playoff opponent

where are the loneliest people

coronavirus latest map and case count

monoclonal antibody treatment

regeneron monoclonal antibody

northern indiana covid infusion center

discovery of virus variant

psalm for healing

recovery rate for people hospitalized with covid

covid hospitalizations recovery rate

recovery from severe covid

covid hospitalizations recovery rate united states

covid pneumonia slow hypoxia

nfl week 17 predictions

coronavirus latest map and case count

covid pneumonia patients who need increased oxygen

covid pneumonia oxygen level that requires ventilator

at what oxygen level is a ventilator needed

is 4 liters of oxygen a lot covid

most rushing yards in a season nfl history

double pneumonia covid
covid pneumonia both lungs
what makes covid 19 go away
what makes covid 19 clear
what makes covid 19 pass
covid pronation
covid proning
antiviral covid
covid what if patient declines ventilator
psalms for healing
wolf pup mummy arctic
mummified penguins antarctica
what if mike pence resigns
coronavirus latest map and case count
how long before symptom onset is a person contagious
coronavirus incubation period
how long does it take for covid to stop being contagious
can you get covid again
covid can you be carrier after recovered
covid clearing lungs
covid does it help to cough up phlegm
how to be safe visiting covid patient in hospital

how safe are hospital ppe masks

how protective is an n95 mask

covid convalescent plasma

covid plasma trial

covid recovery from low blood oxygen

how to recover from low oxygen level covid

gravely ill meaning

things to try when lungs not responding to oxygen

what defines critical condition

plasma treatment covid

covid double pneumonia

end of life visit

how low is blood pressure 89/50

covid and low blood pressure

covid 89 percent oxygen nasal cannula

does plasma help with covid

what allows a serious covid patient to recover

how to survive critical covid

covid ways to heal lungs

covid breathing exercises

covid ards recovery

oxygen bipap

cartoon wonder twins powers activate

end of life oxygen therapy

ipad compare models

side effects using cpap

how to reset ipad to factory settings

heart to heart hospice

center for hospice care elkhart

palliative care

covid hospice care does it work

covid end of life video

covid move from cpap to bipap

mister rogers show about death

mister rogers death of goldfish

catholic readings for funerals

can a mother forget her infant

yes in joy you shall depart

soon and very soon

how great thou art

be not afraid

/

The mother I saw

what I could see of her face
and how she was breathing
behind the mask
was not
from what I could tell
someone who was going
to go home
not someone who was going
to get better
though there was still the Hopkins doc (hope)
and maybe the scan (hope)
and maybe something only he knew (hope)
but my mother
who was awake
but who could not speak
because of the mask
looked for the first time
like someone who really could be
end of life
and that mask

her labored quick inhales

and sometimes a sucking noise it made

I wanted to tear the mask from her face

carry her from the room

to the elevator

and from the elevator to my car

and have her rest her head

on my sister's lap

in the back seat

while I drove her home

where we would lay her in her own bed

and cover her with her own blanket

and her cat might jump up on the bed

for a pet or scratch

and we'd move the digital photo frame

from the kitchen to the bedroom

so that the images of her life

could pass before her eyes

but I knew that without the mask

she would die

I knew this

because on a piece of paper

with the letters of the alphabet
my mother pointed to spell
J-U-I-C-E
and we called the nurse
who came into the room
and removed the mask
and held a small white cup
filled with orange juice
near my mother's lips
but my mother didn't have the strength
or air
to suck the juice through the straw
so we tossed the straw
and held the cup to her lips
one tiny sip
some of the juice dripped onto a towel
my sister held
beneath our mother's mouth
then another careful tiny sip
I looked up to see
that in less than a minute
without the mask

my mother's oxygen had dropped
from 92 to 82
do you want one more sip
(she nodded yes)
only one more okay because—
her oxygen was now in the 70s
she took another sip
and my sister wiped her mouth
then the nurse strapped on the mask
and my mother's oxygen climbed
back into the 80s
then 91-92-93 where it settled
and she slept for a while
my sister holding one hand
me holding the other
then rubbing my mother's feet
reaching behind her to massage her back
touching her face.

/

I forgot to say

that we were living
in a 1950s science fiction movie
before we were allowed in the room
my sister and I put on gowns and gloves
but no need for masks
because we each had our own environment
in which to breathe
a self-respirating helmet
with a plastic shield in front of our eyes
a tube connecting the back of the helmet
to a battery-powered air machine
a small black box strapped to our backs
to keep us from breathing in
the virus our mother was breathing out.
/

Now that we were in the room

we would not leave
not without our mother
not without some kind of answer
a way forward
or word from the doctor
that there was no way forward
or that the only way forward
would not end with our mother home
but would end with her end
here in this room
she slept
and woke to see us there
and slept some more
the respiratory therapist came
to look at her numbers
and at the machine
feeding her oxygen
and said what others had said
that our mother was nearing the limit
of oxygen she could be given

but said let me try one thing
and pressed the machine's screen
and played with the settings
and though we didn't really know
what he was talking about
he said something about the time
between our mother's breaths
and maybe if he changed this one setting
he'd be curious to see
if it had any effect
hungry for hope
we were almost tricked
by this one press of a button
we were waiting to see the Hopkins doc
because the docs at Hopkins
were experts on Covid
and this one
whoever he was
would tell us something
would guide us
would order the scan
so we would know

one way or the other
we held our mother's hand
as she slept
until the doc showed up
he was personable
looked at the machines
the numbers on the machines
then with a stethoscope
listened to our mother's lungs
(he had to move aside one breast
gently
then the other
to listen to her lungs)
he was in the room
(my memory is suspect
we were tired and worried
and wearing what looked like space suits)
around five minutes
then said maybe we should talk outside
so we Hulked off our gowns
threw them away with our gloves
and waited until we were in the hallway

before removing our battery-powered helmets
he said we could do the scan
but I don't think it's necessary
(pause)
she's received all the treatment we can give
and she said no to intubation
which to be honest I think is the right decision
so we've reached that point
where maybe her treatment changes
from healing
to comfort
we asked again about the lung scan
and he said it would be uncomfortable for her
and based on what he was seeing
and the trajectory the illness had taken
in her body
he would not recommend the scan
if she were my mother
he said
I think this would be the time
for comfort
I'm sorry

I know this is hard

my sister and I looked at each other

as if to ask what now

then it became clear

that the next thing to do

was tell our mother

we huddled in the hallway

trying to decide

how to say

what needed to be said

my sister wanted to say

we're going to make sure you're comfortable

they're going to give you morphine

then you can take off that damn mask

but I wondered if our mother would understand

what that meant

my sister said I'm sure she will

and I said but we need to be sure

she has a right to know

and one of the nurses

listening to us

said when you're with your mother

you'll find the right words
or maybe they'll find you
and we put on new gowns and gloves
and our self-respirating space helmets
and went back into the room
my sister on one side of the bed
me on the other
I was the one who spoke
Mom I said
we just met with the doctor
and
(pause)
and he said you're at the max of oxygen
they can give you
and that they've done everything they can
behind her mask my mother nodded
then I had no further words
except
I'm sorry Mom
I'm so sorry
we tried everything
and hugged her

and started to cry
and my sister
who didn't like to see me cry
put her hand on my back
and said it's going to be okay
we'll make sure you're comfortable
we're not going anywhere
not leaving your side.
/

Except I did leave

to tell my father
who had been texting and calling
all morning
and must have been wondering
why no one had responded
when my sister said we weren't leaving
no matter what
she meant we would not leave
our mother alone
at every moment at least one of us
would be with her
I sat in my car outside my father's house
waiting for the right words
and after ten minutes went in
he was sitting where he always sat
in the chair by the kitchen table
I stood six feet away from him
and from behind my mask told him
that there was no chance for her to recover
I said the same words to my father

or similar words
that I had said to my mother
I'm sorry Dad
I'm so sorry to have to tell you this
and he cried a little
and shook his head
and said I knew something was wrong
I just knew
and though my father was Covid positive
I went to him
and put my arm around him
and said again that I was sorry
and that Jen and I would be with her
wouldn't leave her
that she wouldn't be in pain.

/

She was still alive

yet I kept imagining people ask

how old was your mother

in the past tense

when she was not yet

in the past tense

I couldn't help wondering

what people would think

of the number 79

how many years

are enough years

to live

when I search

life expectancy United States women 2020

the CDC tells me: 80.5 years

so maybe

someone might reason

my mother's dying

was expected

right on time

when to me it felt unexpected

too soon

but that life expectancy

is for an American female *born* in 2020

an American woman in 2020

who has *already* reached the age of 75

as my mother had

could expect to live

another 12.9 years

which meant that my mother

could have expected to live

until she was 88

though to be fair

not that life is fair

the life expectancy of a woman

born in 1941

was 70.8 years

in which case

someone might reason

my mother had already lived

eight more years than expected

had lived 36 more years

than her own mother.

/

How old is your mother
was your mother.

/

Rather than a number
it feels better to say
she's the same age as
Ann-Margret
Ryan O'Neal
Bob Dylan
Neil Diamond
Paul Simon
Art Garfunkel
Bernie Sanders
Jesse Jackson
it feels better to say
my mother is Martha Stewart years old
Pete Rose years old
she is Lesley Stahl
Nick Nolte
Beau Bridges
Faye Dunaway years old.

/

I search the names
of people who lived 79 years
Elizabeth Taylor
Johnny Carson
Ella Fitzgerald
John Cage
John Ford
H. G. Wells
Charles Atlas
I want to say that my mother
who is still alive
but dying
will have lived
once her life has ended
as long as these people
about whose lives much more
is known.

/

I didn't want my father to be alone

my brother-in-law came to be with him
then some friends
I stopped at the hotel to eat a granola bar
because I didn't know when I would eat again
then went to the hospital
to relieve my sister
who needed to go home to eat
and check on her daughters
and for the next three hours I was with my mother
just the two of us
she mostly slept
and I held her hand
and rubbed her legs and feet
to make sure she knew I was there
a hospice nurse came in to speak with me
about how the process would work
and my phone
which had to be kept in a clear plastic bag
kept ringing
someone else from hospice on her way

with paperwork to sign
could I meet her in a café
on the ground floor
I told her I wouldn't leave my mother
until my sister returned
and she said no problem
take your time
and as my sister was parking her car
I tore off my gown and pulled off my gloves
and left the room
to find my mother's parish priest waiting
the chaplain had called him
I knew this would be
what my mother wanted
when my sister arrived
she went in with Father Jason
who administered the sacrament of Extreme Unction
anointing of the sick
while I met with the woman from hospice
in an otherwise empty hospital café
half-listened as she put paper after paper before me
to sign

she said I know this is like signing a mortgage
(it was)
I was in a hurry to get back to my mother
still not sure what I signed except
most importantly
consent for hospice care to begin
but two hours later
back in the room
it had not yet begun
my sister and I
whispered to each other from either side
of our mother
wondering *when*
what were they waiting for
and though that may seem odd
to want the process of your mother dying
to begin
the truth was that we did
knowing there would be no recovery
we wanted her to pass in peace
and quickly
though we knew dying took

as long as it needed
sometimes days
and we were ready
exhausted but ready.
/

The first dose of morphine

at 6:45pm
and fifteen minutes later a second
and fifteen minutes later a third
at which point they removed the mask
our mother made a motion
with her closed hands
it looked like she was cheering *hooray*
so glad never to have to wear that mask again
(we would remember this gesture
to remind us that she was ready)
we too felt relief when the mask came off
though we knew what it meant
that it had truly begun
there was no turning back
we were so happy to see her face
that we touched her cheeks
and said Mom your face!
and rubbed her hair
and wanted to take off our rubber gloves
to feel our skin against hers

and to take off our helmets
so that we could kiss her
soon the morphine doses would be stronger
and we knew our time with our mother awake
was short
so together we scrolled through photos
on my sister's phone
and our mother smiled at some
and we even laughed a few times
and I said to my mother
one of the last things I said to her
that I know she heard
I said (touching her arm)
this body / this body
brought us into the world
five minutes apart
and now we're going to shepherd you out
we must have reminded her a dozen times
that we wouldn't leave
we'd be there with her
and then my sister said
soon you'll see your mother

and this

I say with no shame

is what my sister and I believed

that soon our mother would see her mother

for the first time in 65 years

in some way

beyond words

beyond human comprehension

after her mother died

my mother and her aunt moved

some mornings my mother would return

to the building where they used to live

and sit in the hallway

outside their old apartment

until the school bus came

one night she woke from sleep

to see her mother

just for a moment

a ghost / a dream

at the foot of her bed.

/

And though it had already begun

now it truly began
our mother slept deeply through the night
and with each dose of morphine
ever more deeply
her head back
mouth open
snoring the way she'd snore
asleep in her favorite chair
at home
and once I left to use the restroom
and look for coffee
(the hospital seemed abandoned)
and once my sister left
for a break
and we took turns trying to nap
in the recliner
my mother had spent days in
in this room
as long as one of us was by her side
and though it felt wrong

(later my sister would tell me
she was glad I had done it
so that we could remember
what didn't seem real)
I took a selfie
of my sad exhausted face
behind the mask of a science fiction helmet
hours into a new day
in a new year
we had hoped to be better
than the previous
our mother paused more
between breaths
(remember this isn't a poem
though of course the lines
must be broken
because my mother's lungs
were broken
beyond repair
and we must pause for breath
at the end
of each line)

I watched her chest moving
knowing now that her breaths could be counted
(as all of our breaths can be)
and studied her face
and thought for the first time:
I look like her.
/
I dozed off in the chair
and in my sleep had a small seizure
(nocturnal epilepsy)
and woke with a start
to see my sister
resting her head
near our mother's leg
I knew I needed to find coffee
and water
our mother's dying could take
we didn't know how long
I wandered the ghostly hospital
to the cafeteria
where I bought coffee
from a vending machine

and drank it by a window
looking out
into early-morning darkness
and it felt strange and dangerous
to pull down my mask
to sip my coffee
even though I was alone
I used a restroom
washed my hands
turned off the water with my forearm
dried my hands with paper towel
wrapped the wet paper towel around my hand
like a glove
before grasping and turning the doorknob
and pulling open the door
and flipping the light switch
then held the door open with my foot
and tossed the paper towel
into the trash can
I walked along a brightly lit
but empty hallway
stopped in the chapel

to cry

it was easier to cry alone

and I hoped that no one

would walk past and see me

and I hoped that someone

would walk past and see me

and ask are you ok

I prayed that my mother

would remain peaceful

and free from pain

and would be taken soon

though I didn't want her to be taken

anywhere

I rode the elevator back to the sixth floor

to tell my sister to take a break

get some coffee

get out of the room for ten or fifteen minutes

but when I got off the elevator

I saw two nurses see me

and look at each other

and say something to each other

and one of them walked towards me

reached me before I reached the room

and that's how I knew

before she said

I'm so sorry

your mother just passed

I asked if my sister was in the room

and she said yes

and quickly I put on a gown and gloves

and my helmet

with my own private air

and went in to see

my sister holding our mother

our mother as I had left her

head back

mouth open

except not breathing

I hugged my sister

though it's hard to hug

the way you want to hug

hard to fully embrace

when wearing a helmet

and we cried

and then I made sure my mother's eyes were closed
(they were)
and tried to close her mouth
because I wanted her to look
as if she were sleeping
but her mouth wouldn't close
and my sister said
I already tried
it won't close
it's okay
it's normal
and the nurses said we could spend as much time
as we wanted
with our mother's body
and for a while I did what I had done
when she was alive
held her hand
touched her feet
her legs
her arms
her hair
especially her face

my sister told me that she had been resting

her head near our mother's legs

and must have fallen asleep

because silence woke her

the absence of the sound

of our mother breathing

she opened her eyes

looked at my mother

saw that she was still

and said Mom

Mom!

MOM!

and knew

and put her arms around our mother

and held her close

the way she'd wanted to

with no fear she'd hurt her

and stayed that way

just the two of them

rather just the one

now that our mother was gone

and waited five minutes

before calling the nurses

who listened for

but did not hear

my mother's heart

and this is but one story

among millions

and counting

she died

sometimes I say *passed*

sometimes *passed away*

at 5:30am on January 15

which happens to be

we'd discover days later

her mother's birthday.

/

This is not a poem: a reprise

Call it oxygen
if you want
it began with a cough
in the year everyone knew was the worst
we'll never know how
my mother and father
breathed the same air
my sister slept with the phone by her ear
my father could hardly walk
even with his walker
my mother was trembling with chills
at the hospital
they wheeled my mother away
my father couldn't get up
his voice from a great distance
what am I supposed to do
everything became about oxygen
if it's my time it's my time
you know it could get worse
before it gets better

we'll see what happens
nobody knew anything
now we know
we're all going to disappear
one day like a miracle
it's a question of when.
/
I hugged my wife and son
knowing I wouldn't return
the same person
then drove through a long cold
dreary day and night
to see my mother
I leaned over her
reached my arms around her
and through my mask
kissed her head
told her that I loved her.
/
Ridiculous that a son should need to sit
so far from his father
whose wife might be dying.
/

My mother woke one day
hallelujah
with an appetite
and FaceTimed my father
and hallelujah he was so happy
to see her face.
/
Lord let her sleep well
Lord let her breathe better.
/
But my mother had a dark and stormy night
and another
and another
and they gave her morphine
and my sister said
when can you be at the hospital
and the mother we saw
was not
someone who was going home
she didn't have the air
to suck juice through a straw
she slept for a while

my sister holding one hand
me the other
we each wore a helmet
to keep us from breathing in
the virus our mother was breathing out.
/
She slept
and woke to see us there
and slept some more
we wanted her to pass in peace
and quickly
though we knew dying took
as long as it needed
three doses of morphine
then they removed the mask
and there was no turning back.
/
We were so happy to see her face
that we touched her cheeks
and rubbed her hair
we scrolled through photos
on my sister's phone

I said to my mother
this body brought us into the world
now we're going to shepherd you out
and my sister said
soon you'll see your mother
and our mother slept deeply
and with each dose of morphine
ever more deeply
head back
mouth open
pausing more
between breaths
I left to find coffee
wandered the ghostly hospital
used a restroom
stopped in the chapel to pray
rode the elevator back up
and she had already passed
like a miracle
she was gone.
/

Her name was Catherine

same as her mother
most people called her Cathy
my father called her Cat.
/

Last in the room

I was the one to place my mother's belongings
what she had brought with her
on the last day of the worst year
into sealed plastic bags
the shoes she had worn that day
she had expected to go home
her winter coat
pants and blouse
purse
phone
eyeglasses
white rosary beads
the square of paper on which my mother
had spelled J-U-I-C-E
and later D-A-D
to ask how our father was feeling
I set the bags on a chair
because I wanted to touch her again
her hands
feet

legs

arms

hair

and face

but her face

was already growing cold

and that was too much for me

much too much

she was gone

suddenly in sunlight

she was gone

the whole garden will bow

and it was time for me to go.

/

My mother speaks to her children
(in the voice of Teresa of Avila)

I have no body

but yours

no hands

no feet on earth

but yours

yours are the eyes

through which I look

compassion into the world

yours are the feet

with which I walk

to do good.

/

In another version of this story

my mother comes home
lives another x years
but that would mean she'd need
to die again
in some other way
might outlive my father
might need to grieve him.
/
In another version
I would wait longer
maybe much longer
before recording these word-feelings
emotion recollected in tranquility
as Wordsworth said
but Wordsworth also called poetry
(call this what you will)
the spontaneous overflow
of powerful feelings
when Ginsberg wrote about his mother
Naomi underneath this grass

he started on a Saturday at 6am
and with the aid of morphine and meth
and the *strange chemicals* of New York City
completed a draft forty hours later
on Sunday at 10pm
Lord Lord Lord caw caw caw Lord
I wrote this
Catherine underneath this grass
in twenty-five days
same number of days
my mother was sick
still living but dying
dying but still living.
/
In another version
this story would continue
would include the moment we
told my father
that what he knew was going to happen
had happened
another version would include
the woman behind the front desk

at the hotel

saying with midwestern too-friendliness

hey how are you

(my mother just died)

have a great rest of your day

(you too)

and would include the meeting

with the funeral director

who shook my hand

(which I immediately washed)

and expressed his condolences

(his job)

and breathed much too heavily

behind his mask

across the table from me

a binder of coffins between us

and maybe that version would include

choosing two plots in the cemetery

on a bitter cold day

one for our mother

and one beside it

for our father

and writing the obituary
and our meeting with Father Jason
to tell him more
about my mother
because during a Catholic funeral Mass
there is no eulogy
(such as a son would like to give)
only a homily
and that other version of this story
might include the arrival of my wife and son
and the funeral Mass
one hour after Joe Biden became President
twelve people all wearing masks
(except Father Jason)
most of whom had already had Covid
and how light my mother's coffin felt
when we carried it to the hearse
and final prayers at the cemetery
and my son crying
after touching the coffin
and the next day
after two weeks in Indiana

goodbye to my sister and father
and the too-long drive home
and then no more jobs to do
lives to save
or not save
obituaries to write
coffins to pick out
coffins to carry
then: did that really happen
then: what else could we have done
what if we had tried this or that
or done this or that sooner
and me still trying
to close her mouth
still touching her cold face
wanting it to be warm
another version of this story
would go deeper into the grief
as deep as the snow
covering my mother's grave
as I write this
one month after the day she died

as my sister
six hundred miles from here
lays flowers on the snow
above the earth
above our mother's body
another version of this story
would include our first Mother's Day
without a mother
her first birthday
that doesn't age her
her first death day
and the day the stone
which my sister and father chose
is set into the earth
they decided on one stone
my parents would share
one side complete
with my mother's name
and dates of birth and death
the other side with my father's name
and date of birth
but his date of death blank.

/

But I believe
that less is more
unless less
means less life
so let's let this be
whatever it will be
poetry or oxygen
one record of what happened
at the end of the year
people called the worst
and the beginning of the year
people hoped would be better
I will bind this
and rest it upon my mother's grave
until someone takes it
or the wind blows it away
and then I will bind another copy
and another
as many as it takes
until one sinks into the earth
to my mother
I fear she'd read it and say

did this really happen to me
how did this happen to us
but more likely my mother
would read this
and say
it's okay
be not afraid
you loved me this much
to write this
take care of your father
take care of each other
more likely she'd say
others died alone
the faces of their loved ones
on screens
at least my children were with me
at the end
what more could a mother want
and I would say yes
but please don't take my grief
not yet
it's all I have

and she would say
I'm still your mother
I want to protect you
and I would say yes
that's why I need to weep
and she
being the mother she was
would say
though I have no hands
I'm holding yours
and your sister's
and your father's
let's have a good cry
just for a little while
together.
#

Jan. 22–Feb. 15, 2021

ACKNOWLEDGMENTS

my sister
my father
my wife and son
friends and family
too many to name
for prayers and comfort
every nurse and doctor
who cared for my mother
every first responder
every life lost
during this pandemic
and those they left behind.

A NOTE ABOUT THE AUTHOR

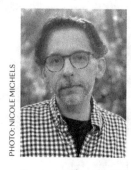

Nicholas Montemarano was born in Brooklyn and grew up in Queens. He is the author of three novels, *The Senator's Children* (2017), *The Book of Why* (2013), and *A Fine Place* (2002), as well as a short story collection, *If the Sky Falls* (2005), which was named a *New York Times Book Review* Editor's Choice. He has published short stories in dozens of magazines including *Esquire*, *Zoetrope*, *Tin House*, *The Southern Review*, *AGNI*, *The Gettysburg Review*, and *DoubleTake*. His nonfiction has appeared in *The Washington Post Magazine*, the *Los Angeles Review of Books*, and the *Los Angeles Times*, among others. His writing has won a Pushcart Prize and fellowships from the National Endowment for the Arts, the Bread Loaf Writers' Conference, MacDowell, Yaddo, and the Edward F. Albee Foundation. He teaches at Franklin & Marshall College, where he is the Alumni Professor of Creative Writing and Belles Lettres.